BYE-BYE DEPLOYMENT, HELLO ENJOYMENT

It Is Never Too Late to Start Living Your Life Again After Deployment

NORMA ELY-JONES

For my wonderful husband, Chris; my family, who is my inspiration, my support, and my rock; and all members of the military who have ever been on deployment—especially those who served in Scania, Iraq—and their spouses and families.

May God continue to bless you.

CONTENTS

INTRODUCTION

Ever since I was a young girl, I was fascinated by military and men and women in uniform. It did not matter whether they were in the Army, Navy, Air Force, or Marines. I liked the way they dressed, saluted, said, "Yes, Sir" and "No, Sir" and generally carried themselves. Therefore, at an early age, one of my dreams was to join the military.

After high school, I went to college and studied business administration. Meanwhile, I still wanted a military career. So, I made the decision to join the Army. I felt that serving my country was a patriotic duty, and for me, it was an honor. The military provided me with an interesting and exciting career along with many opportunities. I travelled, got a chance to grow and develop my potentialities (which included gaining leadership and other skills), and I met people from all walks of life. Some of them remain my best friends.

What I most like about the military is that it instilled in me a desire to give back to others, if only a mere modicum. Some of what the military gave me includes: increased self-esteem, pride, knowledge, wisdom, love for your fellow man, respect and understanding of diversity, and so much more.

I want to share some of my experiences, lessons, and things that blessed and inspired me to want to be a blessing to others. That is why I wrote this book. It is an open and honest sharing of my deployment, the impact of it, and my reintegration into life–the world of work, family, friends, etc. The one thing that I do in this book, and that the military taught me, is to tell the truth, especially when you are trying to help someone, because "the truth will set you free". I want to pass this and other lessons on to you.

I close with the words of an old song that my grandmother used to sing which helped to form my philosophy of life and behavior: " If I can help somebody as I pass along, If I can spread love's message with a word or song, If I can show somebody he [or she] is travelling wrong, then my living will not be in vain".

"Life can only be understood backwards; but it must be lived forward."

\- SOREN KIERKEGARD

One

HAVE YOU BEEN DEPLOYED?

Have you been deployed in one of the military services and are now trying to find some type of normalcy for your hectic life?

When I returned home from deployment in a far-away country that I would never have dreamed of, I did not know the state of both physical and mental desperation I would be in as well as the around-the-clock physical attention I would require daily.

After deployment is over, you don't know what you have been through mentally or physically, because, depending on where you deployed to, there may not have been any mirrors for you to see your body or medical facilities for you to get a checkup.

When I came back to the United States after 180 days in the 120-degrees-in-the-shade desert, I was many shades darker, the front of my hair was blonde, and I weighed thirty pounds more than I did before I left the United States of America's soil.

I looked and felt like a 190-pound stuffed black olive, plus, I was constipated. I know you are dying to find out how I became this way. When I was over in the blazing hot sun, my battalion had the Civil Affairs mission, since no replacement Civil Affairs unit was sent, which meant my soldiers and I had to go out once a month and visit the Iraqi's communities. We had to socialize and eat the food prepared by Iraqi women who used their bare hands as utensils to cook chicken in boiling oil.

Did I mention anything about the fact that they didn't have any running water in their homes? I think you get the picture. I caught a severe case of the Iraqi Crude. I had fluids leaving my body through both exits. The military sick call attendants gave me something to stop the floods, but I didn't know the effects it would have on me in the not too distant future.

Do you just want to get back to where you were before your deployment and continue with your life as before? I did. Before deploying to Iraq, I was one of the most eligible single females in my town. I had a six-figure income, over $400,000 in my savings account, was a perfect size 7/8 dress size, had an officer major rank in the Army Reserves, held a fulltime government job, and built a four-story townhouse with a garage in Northern Virginia.

I know what it feels like to leave everything you hold near and dear, while not knowing if you will ever come home again. I know what it feels like to leave everything you once knew and go across dozens of time zones to foreign lands to serve our country that we hold so dear. I had no idea what I was in for during the eighteen months of my life that would drastically change me. I would never be the same, ever again.

I left all of this behind for deployment to an unknown country with a language I did not speak nor understand, a country where women had no rights and men only wanted male children.

I wasn't married and did not have anyone to handle my affairs, so I had to sell my car, pay off all my bills, rent out my new townhouse, and take a leave of absence from the wonderful job that I was in training for.

I'm talking about all the things soldiers, sailors, marines, and airmen give up to serve our country every day.

When I returned home 180 days later, my townhouse was still rented, so I was homeless for the first time in my life. I didn't have a car because I had to sell the one I had, and the wonderful job I left behind required me to have a medical certificate that I could not get because of the medication I was required to take after returning home.

"Life is a roller coaster. There are ups and downs. There are hills, valleys, and so on. But it's your choice to scream or enjoy the ride."

- MARTEIN LANDEAU MARTIN

Two

THE FEELINGS OF UPS AND DOWNS

I will share with you the feelings of ups and downs, known as post-traumatic stress disorder (PTSD), that occurred after returning from my deployments. My book will offer real-life solutions, suggestions, and experiences that helped me through the uncertainties and medical issues and also helped to save my life and the lives of other soldiers.

I returned from deployment in 2005, and for twelve years, I suspected something was mentally wrong with me, but I didn't understand what it was. I went to dozens of counselors and psychiatrists which cost me a lot of money. Thank God for insurance and the Veterans Affairs Hospital. All of the counselors and psychiatrists talked to me and asked me what I thought was wrong, like I knew what I was going through and was just not fixing it. I told them all, "If I knew what was wrong with me, believe me when I say I wouldn't be here with you."

I filed a claim for PTSD back in 2005 as advised and counseled by one of the VA Doctors. I sought medical attention and was denied. However, a bill was passed in the House of Representatives on July 6, 2011, enacting compensation owed for mental health based on activities in the Theater Post-traumatic Stress Disorder Act or the COMBAT PTSD Act.

The COMBAT PTSD Act was needed, and I'm sure it has helped many deployed military personnel get the care that they so desperately need. When I found out about the COMBAT PTSD Act, I refiled for my combat service-related disability for PTSD, and this time, I *was* awarded it, thank the Lord!

I was happy to be able to go to the Veterans Affairs Hospital in Washington, D.C. to get counseling. I needed to get out of the PTSD maze I had been trapped in for almost fourteen years. I did not care who was in the PTSD groups when I got my counseling. I told the VA counselors that I just needed to talk to someone who could help me find my way back to the way I was before deployment.

I started in a group of about ten other veterans, all men, who had been deployed out of the country and were diagnosed with PTSD and who could relate to what I was going through. The VA counselor was concerned that I was the only female in the group, so I asked her if she had another group with females. When she said no, I told her, "I guess I will be staying in this PTSD group, then." I completed the PTSD group counseling with my ten male military counterparts, and I'm sure we all are better because of it.

During these twelve long years, many of our military brothers and sisters could not bear the ups and downs caused by deployments and have given up their fights for life.

I thought that, once I completed the initial counseling, I was fixed; however, I found out years later that I was wrong.

Over the course of what I will title "that which did not kill me made me stronger" phase in my life, I experienced and went through so much that, had I only known were symptoms of PTSD, I could have prevented. Yet, these were ultimately life changing events that revealed to me that the Lord thought that I was worth saving.

My PTSD symptoms included fear of trust; terminal loneness; emotional regulation; emotional flashbacks; hypervigilance; loss and gain of faith; dissociation; persistent sadness; anxiety and depression; insomnia; and 24-hour heightened awareness. There are many more symptoms that military service members go through after deployment.

It will amaze you to know that I was living without knowing that my mind, body, and soul were all out of synch with each other. They were working at an alarmingly dangerous and heightened state– around the clock.

"*A sum can be put right: but only by going back till you find the error and working it afresh from that point, never by simply going on.*"

- C.S. LEWIS

Three

WHAT ARE THE INITIAL STAGES TO LOOK FOR?

Here are seven things that will help you identify that something is not quite right after you return from deployment:

1. **When you return home from deployment, the only people you want to be with or around are your battle buddies from deployment.** Before you deployed, these were not your bosom buddies, so what are your common denominators? The common denominator is the time you served in deployment together and, usually, that is it. You and your battle buddies may share some sports interests, work for the government, come from the same hometown, or share the same religion.

Please make note of this, because when you start finding your way out of the PTSD maze, you might wonder to yourself, "Why in the hell am I with this person?" It may take you fourteen years to ask yourself that question.

2. **You cannot do anything without your battle buddy, and you are very comfortable being together twenty-four hours a day, seven days a week without stopping or coming up for air.** When family members want to intervene, it is always a problem for you or your battle buddy. You find comfort in the PTSD maze that you do not realize you are in. To better explain it in a term you may be able to relate to, you're in a never-ending, dreamlike, erotic state of mind. Consider what's keeping your relationships alive with your family, friends, and loved ones who are trying to re-connect with you.

3. **You fall in love and marry your battle buddy as soon as you return home from deployment.** This is a no-no. Someone should have slapped and shaken me a couple of times, and maybe even locked my ass up and away from my battle buddy, until I came out of the PTSD maze I was in. I was not in my right state of mind and neither was my battle buddy at the time. WOW!

4. **You spend large sums of money without consulting anyone or seeking financial advice.** A good friend of mine contacted me after I returned home from deployment and said that they had bought into a great investment opportunity in Florida. The great investment deal was for a condo complex that was being built, and I would need to invest $80,000 toward the purchase of a newly-built condo near the PGA golf tournaments. I was told that the investor would have someone

buy it from me before the condo complex was finished based on the market's demand. We all know what happened to the housing market in 2007 and 2008; it took an unexpected nose drive, and everyone got caught holding the bag. I still have that condo today that I cannot sell.

5. **You don't want to engage in activities outside your home.** I was engaging in other activities with my battle buddy (wink-wink) which was why I didn't want to engage in other activities or go out of our house. You may have another reason, especially if you don't have any battle buddies.

6. **You drink more wine and spirits than you did before you deployed.** Piña coladas were our drink when my battle buddy and I returned from deployment because they taste good, and if you put enough rum in them, you can get a decent buzz. The problem with drinking piña coladas is that eventually, you will start gaining weight. We eventually graduated to something stronger to help bury the PTSD maze that we did not know we were in.

When you do this, you do not realize that you're operating each day in a maze and at a heightened state of mind, body, and soul. You are functioning Monday – Friday, if you have a fulltime job, because you're a disciplined military service member and you are always dedicated to the mission. However, on the weekends and when you're on vacation, PTSD is full-fledged, and you don't know it.

There are so many incidents that occurred during this time that I survived through. But, "What does not kill you makes you stronger." Thank You, Lord!

Keep in mind that when you and your battle buddy are always together alone, drinking, everything is all good and dandy;

however, when others come into the maze, all HELL breaks loose. One time we were on a cruise together, and I was invited to take a group picture with my battle buddy, a well-known male comedian, and a female cruiser from the West Coast. I said, "No, I don't want to be in the picture; go ahead." When I realized that the female cruiser from the West Coast was putting her arms around my battle buddy's body, I completely lost my mind, body, and soul. This was the first incident related to the PTSD which plagued my mind, body, and soul.

On another occasion, I was with my good friend celebrating her milestone birthday during a weekend in Hotlanta. We had a wonderful weekend planned, and she had invited me to come and celebrate it with her and a few other select female friends. I begged by battle buddle to come with me, even though he didn't want to come. I did not know that I was in a PTSD maze alongside him, which made me think it was just us against the world. As I stated before, that way of thinking may have been OK without the PTSD, but too much of the wrong spirits caused me to think that others were trying to play in my maze. When I was with the women *without* my battle buddy and partaking in the wrong type of spirits, I was fine, it appeared. But when my battle buddy came around the mix, the hairs on my eyebrows stood at attention. My good friend would tell me, "Girl, don't nobody want your man," however, she didn't know about the PSTD, how the alcohol affected me, and that I didn't want anyone in our maze. Under these circumstances, I cannot elaborate further on this in writing; however, I will tell you more about it, if you ask me.

Here's another example – after thirteen years of it being mostly my battle buddy and me, we were hanging out on the weekends at the Fish Market Watering Hole. I refer to it as the "meat market" due to the activity that I think occurs there. It's not one of my favorite watering holes; however, my battle buddy used to love it, so I would go and endure sheer madness each time we went there. The self-imposed, unknown madness I'm speaking of is the same madness I encountered on the cruise ship. I did not want my battle buddy to look at any other woman besides me, and I didn't want any other woman to touch him. For thirteen years, it was just him and I in our PTSD maze, and I did not want anyone else trying to get into our maze, because I did not play well with others who I thought wanted to play with my battle buddy. That is what too much of the wrong spirits, PTSD, and not having other good friends in your life does to you and your sanity.

One particular Friday or Saturday at the meat market cost me over $20,000 in damages. The Lord got my attention, and I was not harmed physically, only mentally. What I learned from that incident was that drinking too much of the wrong spirits was not doing me any good and was causing me only harm and costing me money that I did not have to give away due to stupidity.

Having the Holy Spirt within me is more important than being under the influence of the wrong spirits, so I, with help from the Lord, corrected one PTSD stressor. Do you know which one?

7. **You have nightmares constantly and are not able to sleep at night.** I wasn't sleeping, which prevented me from being able to operate during the day, which affected my performance at work. Not good. I eventually was prescribed PTSD medicine ten years later to help me get a good night's sleep. It is very hard to return back to work after returning from

deployment because you are expected to operate as you did before you left. You have a job to perform, and nowhere in the human relations regulations does it say anything about helping the deployed military service member get re-acclimated with his or her work alongside any PTSD that they may have encountered. How do you tell your manager that you are dealing with PTSD without possibly jeopardizing your job? Every day for fifteen years now, I have to put on the best act of my life, going to work while in the PTSD maze and operating in a heightened state in order to accomplish the mission in an outstanding manner.

"Fear has never helped anybody make good choices. It leads to clinging when we should be walking."

- HARRIET LERNER

Four

STAYING TOO CLOSE
TO YOUR BATTLE BUDDY

Don't get me wrong; it is important to have a good friend. Shortly (and I do mean shortly) after returning home, I married my battle buddy. We knew each other before deploying to Iraq, but there was no love interest between us to my knowledge. I can only speak for myself.

As I said in an earlier chapter, when I returned home from my eighteen-month deployment, I was homeless for the first time in my life and I did not have a plan. My good ole battle buddy offered his three-bedroom, three-and-a-half bathroom, two-car garage home to live in with him until my townhouse became available again.

Right? No, wrong!

I was suffering from PTSD and so was he, but we didn't know it. We were drawn to what we both experienced in Iraq and what we both had witnessed together for eighteen long months away from our families, friends, and loved ones. We became each other's family, friend, and loved one, and we were not aware that we were making a very big mistake.

I clung to him like white on rice all the time and he never let me out of his sight except for when we were at our jobs.

I had no idea what I was doing by marring my battle buddy. Not a clue. I was aspiring to become a one-star general someday. I had all my checks and balances in order, and I was one-star general material, on course and ready.

All I know is we had a beautiful wedding, went on a cruise for our honeymoon, and didn't let many people into our lives. We were in a PTSD maze and didn't realize it for over ten long years.

Don't get it twisted; we loved each other and still do. We both were suffering from PTSD for fourteen long and not all wonderful years, most of the time without the much-needed treatment that we both desperately needed. My battle buddy husband spent so much of his time helping me with my many medical issues after returning home from deployment in Iraq that he didn't or couldn't seek the medical care that he needed as well until now.

Fourteen years later, I'm now returning the favor to my battle buddy hubby by being here for him through his PTSD maze that he is trying to find his way out of. Iraq was his third deployment, and he has never received any PTSD counseling or treatment of any kind until two years ago. His PTSD maze is more severe than mine. He sometimes sees soldiers that he served with who were killed in action. He goes to PTSD counseling once a week for an hour at the Veterans Affairs Hospital. If he hears sounds like gunshots, it triggers his PTSD.

I had to hide all of the weapons that we have in our house, because he sometimes relapses and thinks that he is in a combat zone and fighting in battle.

I now know that the Lord put my battle buddy hubby and me together fourteen years ago because he knew that we both would need each other after returning home from our deployments to help guide one another through our PTSD mazes.

He took care of me the first ten years after returning from our deployment, and now fourteen years later, I'm returning the favor by being there for him during his PTSD struggles.

"That which does not kill me makes me stronger," and it made our marriage stronger, too. We had a lot of learning to do from our mistakes and the experiences we encountered as a military couple with PTSD, trying to help each other work through it all. We had civilian jobs and a child, and we struggled to keep the faith and be there for each other.

I did not realize that I needed to keep my own stuff separated from my battle buddy's. After thirteen years in the PTSD maze, he started reaching out to other friends from his past.

Once again, The Lord was trying to get my attention regarding the PTSD maze I was in, because I was unaware of it and its impacts. I finally woke up and have realized the errors of the PTSD maze that have been erupting and causing total chaos to my mind, body, and soul for the last fifteen years of my life since returning back home from deployment in Iraq.

"Don't be afraid to ask
Questions. Don't be afraid
to ask for help when you need it.
I do that everyday. Asking
for help isn't a sign of weakness.
It is a sign of strength. It shows
you have the courage to admit
that you don't know something,
and to learn something new."

- BARACK OBAMA

Five

HELP IS ON THE WAY

The first sign of help being on the way was the bill that was passed in the House of Representatives on July 6, 2011, enacting the compensation owed for mental health based on activities in the COMBAT PTSD Act.

Another vital sign is when you're at your VA doctor appointments and the nurse asks, "Are you experiencing any suicidal thoughts or tendencies? Are you thinking about harming yourself or others?"

The first time the VA nurse asked me those questions, I thought, "WOW! The VA doctors, nurses, and administrators asking those questions says to me that someone cares about my well-being and they want to know if I'm experiencing signs of PTSD. They want to help me."

In my quest for help, I found out that there are free programs for veterans that give very valuable and helpful information. I spent most of my time at the VA Hospital and in VA counselors' offices, not having a clue what was wrong with me before I was properly diagnosed with PTSD.

I have very good friends who stayed in touch with me after I returned home, even though I tried very hard to try to dodge them and stay in seclusion with my battle buddy hubby; however, those good friends wouldn't leave me alone. This was what I needed from them. I needed my good friends who I knew before deployment to realize that something was wrong with me and stay in my face as a constant reminder of who I was before I deployed.

I didn't realize that I was in the "I don't want to be bothered" state until ten years later when I was looking up a young lady who I knew before deployment. When I finally located her, she shared with me that I had told her via e-mail that I wanted to be left alone and that I didn't want to talk about my deployment with her. I was shocked and embarrassed that I had acted that way and asked her to forgive me.

This was vital for my battle buddy hubby and me to see our way through the PTSD maze and return to some kind of normality, finally, after fourteen years in the maze.

I trust in the Lord with all my heart, mind, body, and soul, and He has seen me through for fifty-six years and made a way for me to write this book to help make a difference in your life and others' lives, too.

I was born to serve others with a smile in any way that I can. I pray that this book will help me do just that, to help make billions of people smile, too.

I fellowship with other deployed military service members at Shiloh Baptist Church on Duke Street in Alexandria, Virginia, where I serve the Lord on Sundays.

"Now faith is the evidence
of things hoped for,
the evidence of things
not seen."

- HEBREWS 11:11

Six

WHY HAVING FAITH IS IMPORTANT

I have always had a relationship with God from my childhood days growing up in southern Alabama near the coast with my praying Big Mama and Papa. I do not ever remember seeing the Alabama coastal waters as a child. It wasn't until I relocated to central Ohio that I was baptized in a church's baptizing pool some forty-six years later that I had the wonderful opportunity to realize that I can experience God.

I now know that God has been with me all along and has never left me nor forsaken me, ever. Hallelujah!

I'm sure you know, too, that the older some of us get, the closer to God we get. My battle buddy hubby says that we have done all the sinning in our younger days, so as we get older, we realize that we have more days behind us (sinful ones) than we have in front of us (less sin remaining). This means now that we are older, we want to get right with God. This is funny and makes me laugh.

I have always been fearful of the Lord and do my best to abide by
His commandments daily. I am doing much better now that I'm older
(hubby might have a point, right?).

I treat people the way I want to be treated and live by the saying,
"What goes around comes back around to you."

When I returned home from deployment, I prayed all the time,
daily, hourly, and never ceased letting the Lord know how much I
loved Him. It was my love for the Lord that guided me through the
up-and-down-times I suffered.

I could not cross a street by myself. I could not drive alone at night
for a long time. I had to get nighttime glasses for driving, which only
worked when I was looking straight ahead. If I turned my head, I
would become disoriented (not good for nighttime driving). I had a
loss of awareness, anxiety attacks, and nightmares when I slept alone,
and many times when I slept with my hubby. I wake up now when I'm
traveling and don't know where I am at.

Experiencing God has kept me centered and focused on Him and I
can see my way through the PTSD maze to the opening waiting on me
at the end. I experience God through prayer and by listening to the
Word. I listen to Joyce Meyers Monday through Friday while I'm
working out, the late Dr. Vernon McGee on the Bible Bus radio every
morning at 5:50 a.m. on my way to work each day, Pastor Shawn
Thornton and Discovering the Word with Mart DeHaan, and Focal
Point with Mike Fabarez on my way home from work at 3:00 p.m. I
also love to listen to Joel Osteen throughout the day to help me
meditate while I'm driving.

I read the *Daily Bread* Monday through Friday to help educate
myself about the Bible and how the Bible applies to everyday life.

Most importantly, my wonderful hubby and I both love the Lord
and each other and we pray, study, and listen to the word together.

I made it through the PTSD maze. Hallelujah!

I said earlier that The Lord thought that I was worth saving, and He did just that.

Four years ago, after being exposed to the PTSD wave and operating at a heightened state for eleven years with elevated stress levels because of civilian employment triggers and being exposed to possibly unknown chemicals and other unknown health issues from deployment in Iraq for eighteen months, I underwent a double bypass open heart surgery, which I know was of the Lord and helped save my life.

The Lord sent one of my previous supervisors, who I had supervised the year before on my civilian job, to tell me to go and get a full body scan done at the Virtual Physical Clinic in Rockville, Maryland and I listened to him and did just that.

The doctor there told me that I had more plaque build-up in my left main artery for my age than any woman should and asked me if I had been exposed to any chemicals or radiation that I was aware of. I told him about the chemical plant that my Army Logistical Battalion had to remove for force protection at our base camp in Scania, Iraq. He told me to go back to my cardiologist, who I had just seen the Friday before, and show her my CT scans of the 100% blockage in my left main artery in my heart. It is very important to note that I had been seeing this cardiologist for the last five or more years.

Hallelujah! Glory to God!

The Lord thought that I was worth saving, and He did just that. He saved me so that I could help save others by writing this book being a living testimony to all by telling you to go and get a full body scan done as soon as possible to reveal the plaque build-up in your arteries and to keep you and yours from having a heart attack or stroke.

"In family life, love is the oil that eases friction, the cement that binds closer together, and the music that brings harmony."

- FREIDRICH NETZSCHE

Seven

YOU ARE NOT ALONE

I have a loving family who cares about my wellbeing. I'm sure that they were not too happy when I told them that I was deploying to the desert in some foreign land and they would not be able to talk to me or see me again for God only knew how long.

I'm the second girl in a family of two girls and two boys with a fierce, loving, and overprotective mother, and a knows-everybody, just-taking-it-easy father. My mother wanted to talk to someone in charge over the phone, right before I took the bus to go to the deployment station.

I asked one of the sergeant majors I saw standing around to please come to the phone and talk to my mother. She made the sergeant major promise her that he would watch over me and to bring me back home safely. She told him that when he brought me back home safely, she would make him some homemade banana pudding. It is a coincidence that the sergeant major who talked to my mother is the same sergeant major who, after deployment, asked me to marry him and is my battle buddy hubby today.

Others were concerned about me while deployed and sent me care packages that contained creams for my aching feet and letters of comfort and support. My long-lost best friend's loving mother baked me some delicious homemade Johnnycakes and sent them to me in Iraq. I enjoyed them. I normally would share my care packages, but not this time!

When my unit returned to the United States, my mom and dad were there at the re-mobilization station, along with many other families, friends, and loved ones of returning army soldiers.

I was so glad to see my family again and it was a good thing that there was always someone around me for the first two weeks home. Everyone wanted to know everything about me being deployed for the last 180 days and wanted to catch me up on all that I missed as if I had never left. They had no idea what I had been through, experienced, and endured during my deployment. I returned a completely different person.

I am so grateful that the Lord gave me my battle buddy hubby because, without him, I do not know what I would have done. My entire family lives in central Ohio and when I returned from Iraq, I lived in Northwestern Virginia, so I didn't have family members close by to help care for me or for me to live with.

I had very nice people who mentored me on my full-time job as a government worker for thirty-five years, helped me take care of my civilian affairs while I was deployed, and helped me get detailed in a different job when I returned.

"Goodness is about character, integrity, honesty, kindness, generosity, moral courage, and the like. More than anything else, it is about how we treat other people."

- DENNIS PRAGER

Eight

TREATING THOSE YOU LOVE LIKE A MILITARY OFFICER

My battle buddy hubby always had the utmost respect for me as his commander and it never changed once he married me.

My hubby and I talked about how married couples could love each other more and stay married if they would use the military custom and courtesy as their marriage regulation on how to treat their spouse.

In a marriage ministry class presented by Skip and Beverly, directors of the First Baptist Church of Glenarden's Marriage Ministry, I learned the importance of respecting your husband and loving your wife. Skip and Beverly shared with us that when you respect your husband, he will show you love, and when you love your wife, she will show you respect.

Through trial and error, my hubby and I found out that when we are not respectable to one another or show one another love, it sets off our PTSD. After fourteen long years, we have had a lot of opportunities to see the triggers that set off our PTSD and we've had a lot of time to develop ways to be together as a married couple.

Using customs and courtesies in the military is very effective and helps sustain all kinds of personalities and relationships, even after they get out of the military. The customs include the positive action things that are done and the things that you should not do to complement the military procedures required by courtesy.

For example:

1. Never criticize your spouse in public
2. Never offer excuses to your spouse
3. Never turn away from a disagreement
4. Never talk to someone of the opposite sex about your spouse unless they are present
5. Never flip your spouse off
6. Never lie to your spouse (not even a small lie)
7. Always resolve all disagreements before going to bed at night
8. Always respect your husband
9. Always love your wife
10. Always treat your spouse better than you want to be treated

I do not require hubby to refer to me as ma'am and I don't refer to him as sergeant major. He calls me baby and I call him sweetie. The bottom line is the military customs and courtesies have been in existence for over two hundred years, so if it has worked this long, something must be right with it.

My hubby and I truly understand the importance of using these military customs and courtesies as a marriage regulation in our lives since we've returned home, and believe me when I tell you that it works very well for us.

So, why don't you give it a try, too?

"To care for him who shall have borne the battle."

- ABRAHAM LINCOLN

Nine

THE VETERAN AFFAIR'S CRISIS HOTLINE: FRIEND NOT FOE

I usually have a working lunch in my office; however, last Friday I decided to go to our cafeteria because they have wonderful fish on Friday. When I arrived, a group of co-workers and retirees invited me to join them and I did.

One of the men, affectionately called Pinocchio, was telling a story about the experience his walking partner, Joe, and his wife had with the VA's Crisis Hotline. This was his story.

Joe Lewis suffered with PTSD from deployment in Iraq, Bosnia, and Kosovo. He had flashbacks, crying spells, and uncontrolled anger, to name a few of his problems. One night he was running around the house with a gun and a machete threatening to kill anyone who came into his family room, which he called his cave and sanctuary.

His wife called the Veteran Administration's Crisis Hotline for help. When the paramedics came, Joe threatened to kill them. So, they grabbed Joe's wife, ran out of the house, and accidentally locked the door behind them. The wife did not have a key. The paramedics, realizing what they had done by having left an armed suffering veteran alone, called the police. A SWAT team and a lot of uniformed officers showed up with guns blazing, ready to shoot someone. Pinocchio ended the story by telling the group not to contact the Crisis Hotline because they don't know what they're doing and can get somebody killed.

Pinocchio's story provided an "aha movement" for me to reiterate the value of the VA and their services. Thus, I briefly shared the following salient points:

Mission: To full President Lincoln's promise "to care for him who shall have borne the battle, and for his widow, and for his orphan by serving and honoring the men and women who are America's Veteran.

Core Values: Integrity, commitment, advocacy, respect and excellence.

VA Benefits: Disability compensation, pension, education and training, health care, home loans, insurance, vocational rehabilitation and employment and burial.

I stole Pinocchio's audience and told them, "The VA is your friend, not your foe."

The group thanked me for that much needed reminder, and I went on to enjoy my fried fish.

"Life presents you with so many decisions. A lot of times, they're right in front of your face and they're really difficult, but we must make them."

- BRITTANY MURPHY

Ten

ARE YOUR DECISIONS SOUND?

Here are some ways to test yourself to make sure you're on the right track.

1. How much alcohol are you drinking daily?

The worst thing for those of us dealing with PTSD is drinking too much of the wrong spirits. You know it's too much if you are waking up, drinking wine or spirits all day, every day, and passing out and cannot remember a thing. Yes, I call alcohol the wrong spirits, because that's what alcohol is. You know when you've had enough of it when you start acting stupid and can't keep your eyes open. I admit I did some dumb, stupid crap that could have harm myself and others when I was under the influence of the wrong spirits. That's when the Lord got my attention, even in the PTSD maze, and told me, "The Holy Spirit can't stay with you when you consume too many of the wrong spirits, because the Holy Spirit does not like being drunk." I never want the Holy Spirit to ever leave me again. Enough said.

2.   You do not want to return to your civilian workforce.

You are not eligible to retire; however, you don't want to go to work and you are out of annual, sick, and request leave without pay. I know that sometimes the people you work with get on your nerves and they don't respect you or your dedication to deploying. Believe me when I say that I have been working in my civilian job for thirty-five years and served our country for twenty-eight years in the Army Reserves. Some people work in the same government job as me and don't give a damn about me or all that I have done for our country. But remember the saying, "That which does not kill me makes me stronger."

3.   You and your house are a hot mess.

You are depressed and don't know why and you are not seeking help to get out of the PTSD maze you're in. I'm not sure how many years went by when I just didn't care how I looked or how our house looked. I was blessed to have my battle buddy hubby in my life, because he doesn't like clutter or messes, so he kept our house in order. I had a lot of medical issues going on, and I was thirty pounds overweight and hated the way that I looked and felt (remember the 190-pound black olive). I was beyond depressed. I wasn't eating

and that didn't help me lose weight. Do you know how it feels
not to have a bowel movement in over a week or two weeks?
Believe me when I tell you that it doesn't feel good.

4. Every month there is someone new in your life.

You are afraid of a steady commitment and don't know why
you are sabotaging all of your relationships that you want to
keep. I don't have a story for you on this one, because my
battle buddy hubby guarded me like a bulldog guards his
porterhouse steak bone.

Do you have a visual, yet?

5. You are not paying your bills.

Your house is about to be foreclosed on, your car was
repossessed, and you don't care that all of this is occurring. I
have always been responsible for others as well as myself,
because the Lord has provided for me.

When I said that I had a lot of medical issues, I wasn't
kidding you. The Lord provided for my hubby and me
through blessing me with combat service-related disability. I
also told you earlier that I made a not-so-smart decision to
invest in the Florida condo. When the condo was finally built,
I had to purchase it or lose my hard-earned $80,000. I prayed,
applied for VA combat service-related disability without any
assistance, and was awarded the disability for one out of the
twenty service-related injuries I submitted my VA claim for.
The Lord provided for me to make the over $2,000-a-month
condo payment and over $300 condo association fees.

6.   **Your friends keep inviting you to church.**

You believe in God; however, maybe when you were deployed something happened that made you lose your faith and hope. I attended church every Sunday morning while deployed in full LBE gear and with a Glock 45 millimeter strapped to my thigh. The Lord told me that everything would be okay when was I sent away from the Iraqi Air Force Base to an abandoned truck stop out in the middle of nowhere to operate a logistics convoy support center with little support. For 180 days, I operated on faith and faith alone, because my faith in the Lord brought my soldiers and me home.

ACKNOWLEDGEMENTS

I thank and praise my heavenly Father, my Lord and Savior Jesus Christ, for all that He has done for me, especially during my deployment and what He does each day.

I thank my buddy hubby, Chris, whom I love and adore because he means the world to me.

I thank Dr. John Shamley and his daughter Benefsheh (Bam Bam) Verell, author of *Military and Mindful,* who introduced me to Dr. Angela Laurin, CEO of Author Incubator, and her staff who helped me to start writing this book; and I thank Dr. Catherine Williams of STEPS Publishing and her staff who helped me to finish it.

I thank the 55th Material Management Command in Fort Belvoir, VA for selecting me to involuntary transfer to the 300th Aerial Support Group to deploy with their group as the supply service officer.

All of you contributed to helping me to write this book which will help make a difference in the welfare and happiness of deployed or undeployed service members' lives.

Thank You!

ABOUT THE AUTHOR

Norma Ely- Jones is a multi-talented retired U.S. Army veteran with an impressive track record for serving our country and working for the Federal Aviation Administration (FAA).

During her twenty-eight years of service in the Army, Norma specialized in quartermaster/logistics and monitored the educational and career tracks of soldiers under her command. She commanded a battalion in Iraq from 2003-2005 and was awarded the Bronze Star. Her last command was as a brigade commander at the 206th Regional Support/ Brigade (Springfield, Illinois). Upon her retirement from the U.S. Army on September 26, 2013, she was awarded the Legion of Merit for her outstanding service.

Norma simultaneously worked for thirty-five years as an air traffic controller for the Federal Aviation Administration. She was the first African American female to hold the position of air traffic manager for the Andrew Air Traffic Control Tower, the primary airport of the President and Vice President of the United States, their families, and dignitaries. She is currently the FAA south team manager in the Air Traffic Services, Technical Advisory Group. She was inducted into the Asian American Government Executive Network's (AAGEN) 2019 Senior Executive Service (SES) Development Program.

Her education background includes a Bachelor of Arts in Aviation from Florida Memorial University, where she was given a Lifetime Achievement Award and inducted into the Historically Black Colleges and Universities Alumni Hall of Fame; and a Master of Business Administration from Strayer University.

Norma has a loving, caring spirit and gifts of counseling and serving which she uses to mentor coworkers, high school and college students, and members of Shiloh Baptist Church where she serves in the Senior Usher Ministry and utilizes other spiritual gifts: administration, giving, and helps. She gives God all the glory for what He has done and continues to do in her life.

THANK YOU

I thank you for taking time to read this book. I have a heart for all individuals in the military serving our country–especially those deployed and returning home.

Please know that I am here to help you survive and thrive as functioning civilians. I provide: personal and career counseling; information and referral services; help for obtaining appointments; monitoring, tracking, and follow up.

If you want to understand more about how I can help you, please contact me:

Facebook: facebook.com/NormaEly/
Twitter: twitter.com/NormaElyJones
Instagram: instagram.com/NormaElyJones
LinkedIn: linkedin.com/NormaEly

I look forward to hearing from you.